THE ULTIMATE GUIDE TO THE PA SCHOOL INTERVIEW

MARK VOLPE, PA-C

BRIAN PALM, PA-C

THE ULTIMATE GUIDE TO THE PA SCHOOL INTERVIEW

1st Edition

ISBN-13: 9798878638418

Published by Kindle Direct Publishing, Charleston, SC

ABOUT THE AUTHORS:

Mark Volpe, MPH, MMSc, PA-C is a Physician Assistant practicing in outpatient internal medicine and urgent care in Connecticut. He graduated from the Yale University PA Program in 2015. He completed his MPH from Southern Connecticut State University and his BS from the University of Connecticut. He has a particular interest in PA program admissions, education, and physician assistant research. During and after his time at Yale, Mark has been published in several peer reviewed journals, served as a special advisor to the BHSc program at Southern Connecticut State University, and guest lectured in local PA program public health and clinical medicine courses. He has served on the admissions committee of the University of Saint Joseph PA Program in West Hartford, CT and has extensive experience interviewing PA candidates. Additionally, Mark precepts students from Yale University and is the former author of the best-selling *Applicant's Manual of Physician Assistant Programs*, now on its 8th edition.

Brian Palm, PA-C is a Physician Assistant practicing aesthetic medicine in the Atlanta, Georgia area. He graduated from the South College PA program in 2013. He also completed his BS from the University of Tennessee. He is well known for his personal statement editing service, myPAresource, through which he helped thousands of applicants gain admissions into PA programs. He was also instrumental in developing the Pre-PA student membership in collaboration with the American Academy of PA's, and previously ran a nationally acclaimed Pre-PA Conference every year attended by thousands of prospective applicants. He has worked with several PA program admissions committees throughout the country and brings his wealth of knowledge and experience to this endeavor.

PREFACE:

We are very excited to bring you the first edition of *The Ultimate Guide to the PA School Interview*. We hope that this resource will be an asset in helping you prepare for your PA interviews.

We have collaborated with PA faculty from throughout the country to make this the most comprehensive interview prep book that is on the market. In this book, you will find everything you need to tackle the PA school interview with confidence that you can be successful in gaining admission to PA school.

Throughout the book we will review various components of the interview including:

1. Program Overview
2. Campus/Facility Tour
3. Questions to Ask Current Students
4. Traditional Interview Questions
5. Situational Interview Questions
6. Ethical Interview Questions
7. MMI Interview Questions
8. Group Interview Questions
9. The Interview Writing Sample

We wish you the best of luck in your journey towards becoming a Physician Assistant!

Best,

Mark Volpe, PA-C
Founder, *The Applicant's Manual of Physician Assistant Programs*

Brian Palm, PA-C
Founder, *myPAresource*

FOREWORD:

Welcome to the journey towards becoming a Physician Assistant (PA)! For more than 10 years, I have been helping students gain insight into the application process to help them get accepted to PA school. After speaking at multiple pre-PA clubs, conferences, and events for those interested in becoming Physician Assistants, the preparing for the interview can cause some serious anxiety.

The decision to pursue a career in healthcare is a commendable one, and your interest in joining a PA program is an exciting step forward. As a practicing PA, I understand the anticipation and nerves that come with the interview process. Therefore, I am honored to share some insights and encouragement as you embark on this crucial phase of your academic and professional endeavors.

The interview process for PA school can be both exhilarating and daunting. It's a time when you have the opportunity to showcase your passion for patient care, your dedication to the profession, and your readiness to take on the responsibilities of a healthcare provider. But it's also a time when you may feel the pressure to perform your best and stand out among other qualified candidates.

First and foremost, remember to be yourself. Authenticity is key during the interview process. Admissions committees are not only evaluating your academic achievements but also seeking candidates who demonstrate empathy, communication skills, and a genuine desire to serve others. Reflect on your experiences, both personal and professional, that have shaped your decision to pursue a career as a PA. Share your unique perspective and what sets you apart from other applicants.

Preparation is crucial. Take the time to thoroughly research the PA programs to which you are applying. Familiarize yourself with their mission, values, and curriculum. Be ready to articulate why you are drawn to each specific program and how it aligns with your career goals. Practice answering common interview questions and consider participating in mock interviews to gain confidence and polish your responses.

During the interview, remember to listen actively and engage with your interviewers. Be prepared to discuss current healthcare issues, ethical dilemmas, and the role of PAs in today's healthcare landscape. Show enthusiasm for lifelong learning and professional growth. And don't forget to ask thoughtful questions that demonstrate your genuine interest in the program and your future as a PA.

Finally, regardless of the outcome, approach the interview process as a learning experience. Each interaction provides valuable insights and opportunities for growth. Whether you receive an acceptance letter or face disappointment, remember that the journey towards becoming a PA is a marathon, not a sprint. Stay resilient, keep striving for excellence, and trust that the right path will unfold in due time.

I wish you the best of luck as you navigate the PA school interview process. Embrace the challenges, celebrate your accomplishments, and never lose sight of the impact you will make as a future healthcare provider.

Brian Palm, PA-C
Founder, *myPAResource*

TABLE OF CONTENTS

CHAPTER 1: THE BASICS

INTRODUCTION

Congratulations! You landed yourself your first PA school interview. You are probably experiencing many emotions right now including joy, happiness, fear, nervousness, excitement, and anxiety. After all this is what you've been preparing for the last several years of your life and now you finally have a chance to show the admissions committee why you should be whom they accept into their PA program.

Before we get into the details of the interview itself, we wanted to give you insight and perspective on what happens behind the scenes before the interview. Once you apply to PA school, the schools which you applied to receive your application and score it. Each school gives a different number of points to the various components of your application including your academic record, your clinical experience, your volunteer experience, your letters of recommendation, your personal statement, and any other noteworthy aspect of your application. Each program is different in how heavily they weigh each of these components, but ultimately nearly every program has a scoring matrix that they utilize to ensure fair, unbiased admissions practices. After scoring your application the admissions committee will review the scores of the applicants to the program and select those that either meet a program specific cut off score or fall within the top 10 to 20% of overall applicants for interviews.

A similar process also occurs after the interview. The admissions committee will score your interview based on program-specific standards and then generally will combine your interview score with your application score to come up with an overall score that will be used to determine who is admitted into the program. In addition, if there are any red flags that come up during the interview process these will be noted and a candidate may be disqualified from consideration. Students will generally either be accepted, waitlisted, or rejected outright at this point.

COMPONENTS OF THE INTERVIEW DAY

Believe it or not, a lot more happens on the interview day than just the interviews themselves! In this section we will review the basics about different types of interviews you may experience, but also the other components of interview day.

▶ Program Overview

Most programs start off the interview day with a program overview. This is usually a short lecture which is given by one of the faculty members or the program director to familiarize yourself with the program. They may review the didactic portion, the clinical portion, any research portions, and anything that really makes the program stand out or makes it unique. Remember, it is their job to sell their school to you as a prospective student and your interview day is as much about them getting to know you as it is you getting to know them. During this time it is definitely recommended to take notes on things you may not have known about the program and think of possible questions you might be able to ask during the interview process if you haven't already thought of those ahead of time.

▶ Campus Tour

Additionally, most programs will also provide a tour of the facilities and perhaps a tour of the entire campus as well. Usually, these tours are given by students that are currently in the program, so this is a great time to ask any questions you may have about the program that you may not feel comfortable asking to a faculty member and really to get an insider perspective on the program itself. Still, it is important to remember to act professionally and courteously during this time as the students can and will report back to their faculty members if there are any red flags that pop up. It might be a good time to ask them about a typical day in the program, or what their study schedule is like.

▶ Individual Interview

The individual interview is a one-on-one interview between you and a faculty member. Sometimes programs will replace faculty members with alumni, current students, clinical preceptors, or members of the community. Of course, if you're not interviewing with the faculty you will have to tailor your answers somewhat to who is interviewing you. These can last anywhere from 10 to 30 minutes on average and sometimes you will have multiple individual interviews throughout your interview day. Most commonly, traditional interview questions are asked during the individual interview. Sometimes the interviewers are blinded to your application (meaning they have not yet reviewed it) to eliminate any biases they may have or to foster learning more about you as a person rather than simply discussing your application.

▶ Group Interview

During this interview a faculty member or group of faculty members will typically interview a group of potential candidates at the same time. They may ask the same question or questions to each candidate or they may ask a single question to one candidate and then build off of that and ask different questions to the other candidates. This is an opportunity for them to see a little bit of your personality and how you interact with your future colleagues. It's important to not be overly aggressive, but also to make sure that you take some time to speak and let your voice be heard as well.

▶ Multiple Mini Interviews

Multiple Mini Interviews (MMI) are short 5 to 10 minute interviews that can happen with faculty members, staff, alumni, or other community members. Most often they are scenario based and you will be given a scenario prior to entering each room that you either have to act out or respond to. Sometimes the interviewer will also ask follow-up questions, while other times they are intentionally mute and simply there to observe your behavior and responses. Usually, programs will have six to eight stations that students will cycle through. Topics can include ethical questions, patient scenarios, behavioral questions, critical thinking exercises, problem solving exercises, and others. Programs will sometimes use a station to get a writing sample as well.

▶ Panel Interview

In a panel interview two or more interviewers will interview you as a prospective student. Sometimes this is done just so that multiple faculty members can meet each student and ask them questions. Sometimes this is done because faculty members will play various roles such as "good cop, bad cop" and they are looking to see how the prospective student reacts. These interviews can be very intimidating because you are outnumbered, but it is important to keep your composure as this is most often one of the major things they are evaluating during these types of interviews. Try to engage with all of the panel members and make good eye contact. Question topics can vary for these interviews, but often do include questions from your application.

▶ Virtual Interview

The virtual interview is an interview day that is held over videoconferencing or over the phone. They can include all the same components of an in-person interview. These interviews became more popular during the COVID-19 pandemic and some programs are beginning to permanently adopt them. The nice thing is that you don't need to travel to these interviews so you can save quite a bit of money on travel costs and lodging. Of course, the downside is that you don't get to visit the program itself and there is something to be said about stepping foot on a program campus and getting a feel for what it is really like to be a student there.

It's important to treat this like any other interview, even though it is virtual. You should still dress professionally and present yourself as you would if the interview were in person. It is also important to set yourself up for success in advance of the interview itself. You should check your laptop and your technology ahead of time and make sure that you have a strong internet connection, a functioning camera, and the appropriate software installed on your computer. You can even try out the interview platform in advance with a friend or family member to make sure that it works on your computer. In a pinch, it is ok to use a smartphone instead of a computer but note that the image quality will not be as good and it's possible that your interview could be interrupted by a phone call or a text message. It is okay if everything does not run smoothly during the interview. Interviewers know the technological difficulties happen, and generally will not hold it against you if you made your best effort to remedy the situation and plan in advance.

In addition, you should make note of your surroundings for the interview. Ideally you should be in a quiet, well-lit room with a neutral background such as a blank wall or window. Anything that is seen in your background is fair game for interviewers to ask questions about and may take away time from your more important interview questions. It is important to rid yourself of any distractions and to turn off the television, cell phone, Apple Watch, any computer notifications, any alarms, and make sure that there will not be any interruptions during your interview. Ideally, you should use headphones during your interview for a more quiet, private environment.

▶ Group Activity

Many programs utilize a group activity as a means of getting to know the applicants better period typically this will involve a puzzle or word problem or critical thinking question that the group needs to work together to answer or to solve. The admissions members will simply observe and typically will not engage with the group until the end of the exercise at which point, they may ask follow-up questions on the exercise. They are looking to see what personality traits you have, who is a leader, who is a follower, who is a problem solver, who is a peacemaker, and how these personality traits would impact your ability to work as a member of the health care team. They are also looking for any red flags such as applicants being dismissive of other people's ideas, getting frustrated or rude with other group members, or excluding others from the activity. One classic group activity is having a small group of students sit in a room and given a prompt that states only one of the students in the room can be accepted into the PA program. The group will have to come to a consensus as to whom should be accepted and why. In general, faculty members are more so interested in the process rather than the outcome for these types of activities.

▶ Writing Sample

Some programs utilize a writing sample during the interview process. The writing sample is utilized for several reasons. Firstly, they want to see if you can synthesize and analyze a situation, form an opinion, and articulate your thoughts. Secondly, they simply want to see if you are a competent writer. They know that many times personal statements and supplemental application responses are reviewed by essay editing services, family members, friends, advisors, and others. Thus, they want to see how well you can write in the moment, unassisted. Finally, they may use the essay as an ethical scenario that they would like you to respond to. This is to your benefit because it gives you a chance to really think about the scenario and put together your thoughts before responding, unlike a traditional interview where you may only have a few seconds to think about the scenario and reply. Overall, you should write enough to answer the question thoroughly, nothing more and nothing less.

▶ Exams

Occasionally, programs will surprise applicants with an exam during the interview. The purpose of this is really to see how you respond under stress more than it is to see what your knowledge is on a particular topic. Questions may involve anatomy, physiology, medical terminology, math, English, or other topics to throw you off. Again, this should not dramatically affect the outcome of your interview day. Just make sure to complete the entire quiz as best you can.

▶ Meals

Oftentimes breakfast or lunch are supplied by programs at the interview. Usually this is a time where the program will have current students sit with applicants to get to know them better and to answer any questions they might have. Though it is not a critical component of the interview, this is a time where you can get important questions answered that you feel more comfortable asking to students. Again, as stated previously, students will pick up on any red flag behaviors and report these back to the faculty members. Even though you may not be scored during this part of the interview, the student input is taken into consideration, and you still want to present yourself professionally and as someone who they would want as a classmate. If you avoid doing or saying anything inappropriate, you have nothing to worry about.

GETTING READY TO INTERVIEW

▶ Practicing for Interviews

In general, the most important thing you can do to prepare for an interview is to practice. Family and friends are reasonable resources you can use to practice your interview technique and know that they certainly aren't experts in the field and may not be able to provide the best feedback. Still, having an opportunity to practice reciting your answers to the most common questions in front of an actual human being can really be helpful to see where you may be stumbling or maybe falling short. In general, it is highly recommended to practice answering questions out loud, even if you are by yourself. By doing this, you will be more comfortable on interview day.

Another common resource for interview practice is your university Resource Center. Many universities will have a premedical or other type of office that offers free mock interviews for students that are applying to professional schools. These are a very good resource and again another set of eyes and ears to hear answers to the most asked questions at these interviews. Certainly, they may not know the specifics of applying to PA school, but they can definitely give you good guidance on your answers as well as simple things like your posture and your eye contact and your overall appearance during the interview process that can definitely be helpful.

Finally, if you are very nervous about your interview or really looking to be as prepared as possible, another option is scheduling a mock interview. There are many companies that offer mock interview services for students who are applying to PA schools, and these are generally individuals who were previously faculty members at PA programs or who have experience in being involved in the admissions process at PA programs. They can get pricey, but if you think of it as an investment in your future and you really feel as though you need the help, it can totally be worth it. We recommend *The Posh PA* (Michele Neskey, PA-C), for all your mock interview needs. There are several other reputable services as well.

▶ *Researching Schools*

Before going in for your interview it is important that you do your research on the school you will be interviewing at. One of the best resources for reviewing the details of any PA Program in the United States is *The Applicant's Manual of Physician Assistant Programs* (Mark Volpe, PA-C and Brittany Hogan, PA-C). This can be useful before you apply to programs, as well as when you are researching programs for your interview.

In general, there are a few things to focus on when researching programs. Firstly, you want to take a look at the program's mission statement. Mission statements can vary significantly from program to program with some programs having a focus on underserved patients, primary care, surgery, leadership, research, or innovation. You want to make sure that your values and what you are looking to get out of your PA program are aligned with their values. It is very common during the interview process to be asked about the mission statement and why or how it resonates with you and you will want to have good reasoning for why you applied to that particular program and how it resonates with you and your life experiences.

Secondly, it is important to review the program website. You want to have a solid understanding of the curriculum of the program as you don't want to be asking questions during the interview that easily could have been found out from the website. It's also important to notice if there are any features that make the program unique, because these are items that you could bring up during the interview as reasons for why you want to attend that program. For example, some programs may offer international rotations, a research curriculum, an addiction medicine rotation, or something else special that will really make the program stand out. Faculty like to know that you have done your homework, and this is one way to show that you did.

Finally, in addition to reviewing all of the available information about the program itself, it is important to actually sit down and review your application (and supplemental application) before the interview. It may have been many months since you last worked on your application and it's important to have good knowledge of exactly what you put on your application as your application will likely be a source for questions from faculty members during the interview process. You want to be able to expand on the experiences, leadership roles, research, awards, and other information you may have supplied on your application and what you took away from it that has helped you in your journey to become a PA.

▶ Attire

One of the most overlooked components of the interview is your attire. Having been on several different admissions committees, I can tell you that there are almost always comments about applicant appearance, clothing, jewelry, and tattoos. Generally, the comments are negative. No one notices the person who is wearing the standard blue or black suit, dress shoes, simple earrings, or necklace. No one notices the person who is well groomed, who has neatly trimmed facial hair, or who is wearing simple makeup. As far as your attire goes, that should be your goal: to not be noticed. You don't want to stand out from the crowd as it can be distracting for the people who are interviewing you or could be seen as unprofessional. For men, the standard blue, black, or gray suit and tie are expected. For women, a pant suit or skirt suit are expected. This is not the time to make a statement with your clothing choice.

▶ *Financial Preparation*

Another commonly overlooked aspect of the interview process is the cost of interviewing. There's nothing worse than when an applicant receives an interview but financially is not able to go because of cost considerations. Applying to PA school is expensive. Just the common application itself and supplementals can cost you thousands of dollars depending on how many programs you are applying to. Once, you receive an interview you may have to pay for flights, hotels, rental cars, food, and other necessities for your trip. In addition, if you don't have a suit that is suitable for interviewing you may have to purchase one of those as well and they can be expensive.

After the interview, you also must consider that you will likely have to pay a seat deposit to hold your spot in the program if you are accepted. These can range anywhere from $500 to $2000 at most programs, and they generally are nonrefundable meaning that if you decide not to attend that program in the future you will not be able to get your money back. You should do your best to make sure you have money available to cover all these expenses. Additionally, if you qualify, make sure to apply for the CASPA fee waiver, or any standardized test fee waivers that may be available.

▶ Interview Day

Once you have received an interview, you are probably wondering what to expect on interview day. Although this can obviously vary from program to program, there are typically three major components to the interview. The first component is usually a program overview. During this a faculty member or perhaps program director will review the basic components of the program including the didactic curriculum, clinical curriculum, and any other unique features for the program. This information is likely also found on the program's website, but if you learn something new be sure to jot it down as it may be something you could bring up in your interviews later in the day.

The second component of the interview is generally a tour of the campus or tour of the PA program facilities. During this they will take you to the didactic year classrooms, study spaces, student lounge, anatomy lab, physical exam suite, and any other places that you may utilize on campus such as a cafeteria, gym, or library. Typically, these tours are led by current PA students so it's a great time to get to ask them any questions you might have about their program, study schedule, school-life balance, or anything else that is on your mind.

The final and most important component of course is the interview itself. The interview format varies by program but can include individual interviews, group interviews, MMI interviews, a panel interview, a group activity, a writing sample, behavioral or situational questions, quizzes, or a question and answer session. Programs will often provide information about the interview in advance of the interview to the applicants. You can also oftentimes find out information about the interview process at certain programs by reviewing their website, searching the PA forums, or searching through social media groups such as The Pre-PA Club on Facebook. In general, if the program does not provide much information about the interview, it is intentionally done so that no applicant has an advantage over another and to see how you respond to a less predictable situation.

▶ What to Bring

The most important thing to bring to the interview is yourself. You want to be on time to the interview, at all costs. You should plan to be at the interview site at least 30 minutes to one hour before the interview is going to start. This way you won't have to worry about any traffic jam, late Uber driver, spilling your coffee on your clothes as you are running out the door, or any other small thing that could make you late to the interview. Plus, when you arrive early this gives you an opportunity to calm your nerves, get comfortable in the surroundings, run through interview questions or major points that you want to make at the interview in your head, and give yourself a pep talk before heading in.

There are some other things that might be helpful to bring as well. It is always advisable to praying a pen and paper with you in the form of either a professional notebook or folder. You can use this to take notes during the program information session and also can write down what questions you would like to ask the faculty members at the program in advance so that you don't forget. You can also bring a copy of your application to review if you have any downtime and also a copy of your resume to review or provide to faculty members if requested. Bringing a small water bottle or beverage is also a good idea, in case your voice gets hoarse or you just want something to sip on during the day. Overall, it is always better to be overprepared rather than underprepared.

▶ Brainstorming

One of the most important exercises you can do prior to interviewing is brainstorming. Simply thinking about events in your life that were either critical moments that led you to pursuing the PA profession or in some way really impacted you, can give you fodder when trying to answer difficult questions on interview day. Ideally during your interview what you can do is use these stories to illustrate certain characteristics about you that you would like the interviewers to know before you leave. These stories could be example from work experiences, patient care experiences, college, personal illness, family illness or tragedy, or anything else that you learned a lesson from or that illustrates important character attributes. This allows you to "show" them who you are rather than "tell" them who you are, and enables them to form a deeper connection with you as an applicant. You should think about what are the three or four things that you want your interviewers to know about you before you leave and come up with ways to incorporate them into your answers to their questions on interview day.

▶ Final Tips

It is important to remain positive during the interview process. You may feel as though you didn't answer a question as best you could but you need to move on and stay positive so that you can continue to perform well during the rest of the interview. Doing something as simple as smiling can really make a difference during the interview.

You should also strive to be yourself and to be honest. You want to avoid the cookie cutter answers to the common traditional questions that are asked at PA school interviews. I once had a faculty member tell me that if an applicant in responding to the typical question of why you want to be a PA said "I like science. I enjoy working with people. I can make a lot of money as a PA" that they would accept them in a heartbeat because it would be the most honest, refreshing answer that they would have ever received to that question. Though these may not be your reasons for pursuing the PA profession, you don't need to make it overly complicated, or tell them the answer you think they would want to hear.

You should practice saying your answers out loud and recording yourself with a camera. In doing so, you will learn about any bad habits you might have when speaking including using filler words, fidgeting, avoiding eye contact, abnormal posture, and anything else that might seem annoying to the interviewer that you can correct in advance of the interview. It also helps to practice saying your answers out loud so you can listen to the way that you answer questions afterwards to really refine what you want to say and how you want to say it. Avoid saying "Physician's Assistant" at all costs.

It's also important to be okay with silence during the interview. You may be able to answer a question very quickly and easily. You don't need to feel as though you need to come up with more things to say just to fill the time. It is also okay to pause after you are asked an interview question and think about it for a few seconds before responding. Again, silence is okay, and you don't want to just blurt out the first thing that comes to mind because it may not be the best answer to the question you were asked. Instead, faculty members will appreciate you giving their question some thought before responding.

Finally, stay on topic. It is easy to get sidetracked during interviews, especially when you come in with an agenda of what you would like to say in advance of the interview. It's great that you have prepared, but always make sure to answer the question at hand first and foremost.

CHAPTER 2: TRADITIONAL INTERVIEW QUESTIONS

INTRODUCTION:

In this section, we will review the most common interview questions that you will be asked. These generally fall into the traditional questions category and are predictable. Although the entire interview will likely not consist of this type of questions, almost all interviews do include these in some form. for the top questions, we will also review the major pitfalls that you should avoid when answering the questions to set yourself up for success. Finally, we will include some additional questions for you to think about and prepare answers for on your own.

THE TOP 5 QUESTIONS

1. Can you tell me a little bit about yourself?

This question is asked by most interviewers as a simple icebreaker. Sometimes they will review your application in advance and so they will already know a fair amount about you, but in a blinded interview they may not know very much about you. This is the opportunity to highlight certain things about yourself or your application that might be interesting or that you might want them to remember about you when considering you for admissions.

The first thing you should do in answering this question is simply introduce yourself. State your name and where you are from. You may even want to consider a handshake or other welcoming gesture as well. Next, you want to tell them a little bit about your background. Some things you could include are where you grew up, where you went to college, your major field of study, or your current job in the medical field. Afterwards, you will want to add any hobbies or interests you have whether they are medically relevant or not. The key here is hopefully to have something memorable about yourself that the interviewer can recall when considering you for admissions. You could talk about clubs, sports, research, mission trips, traveling, pets, or anything else that is an important part of your life. Finally, have a conclusion, such as "I'm excited to be here today".

There are also several things that you should avoid when answering this question. Firstly, this is not the time to talk about why you want to be a PA or what a PA is. You will have time to do that later on in the interview when that question is asked. Secondly, this is not the time to ask any questions about the program that you might have. There will be time for that at the end of the interview. Thirdly, avoid jumping into why you are a great fit for their program. You will have ample opportunity to demonstrate that when answering other questions.

To recap:

Do
- Introduce yourself
- Talk about your background
- Discuss your hobbies, interests, and anything else that makes you unique

Don't
- Discuss why you want to be a PA
- Ask questions about the program
- Talk about why they should accept you

2. Can you describe what is a PA?

There is no hidden agenda with this question. The faculty generally just want to know that you have done your research on the profession, and you have an idea of what the role of the PA is on the medical team. You do not need to make this answer overly complicated.

There are several definitions you can look to for inspiration. The American Academy of PAs definition of a PA is "PAs (physician associates/physician assistants) are medical professionals who diagnose illness, develop and manage treatment plans, prescribe medications, and often serve as a patient's principal healthcare provider. With thousands of hours of medical training, PAs are versatile and collaborative." Another definition comes from the Physician Assistant Education Association, which defines a PA as "PAs are medical providers, most with graduate-level educations. They are licensed to diagnose and treat illness and disease and to prescribe medication for patients.". Finally, the National Commission on the Certification of PAs defines a PA as "PAs are highly qualified, licensed members of health care teams that diagnose and treat patients, prescribe medications, assist in surgery and more. PAs are educated in the medical model and undergo periodic assessments of medical knowledge and continuing medical education throughout their careers."

As you can see, these definitions are more similar than they are different and there are several key components you want to include when answering this question to a faculty member. You should include that PAs are medical providers. They can diagnose, order and interpret tests, prescribe medication, and practice in almost any field. They work in collaboration with physicians and the healthcare team. They are highly trained. In addition, after stating the basic definition, you should try to connect your experiences with PAs from either shadowing or work to the definition. Talk about what you have personally seen PAs do for patients and the relationships you have seen with PAs and the members of the healthcare team.

There are a couple things to avoid as well. You want to make sure that you're using the correct terminology. Most PAs prefer the term collaboration rather than supervision to describe their relationship with physicians. Additionally, terms like mid-level provider or advance practice provider are generally seen as somewhat derogatory by many PAs. The term mid-level provider implies that we only provide mid-level care, rather than high level care. The term advance practice provider lumps us in with nurse practitioners, who are trained very differently from us PAs. It is best to avoid these terms when describing what a PA is during your interview. Finally, make sure you do not say "physician's assistant" during your answer or the interview. PAs are not the property of physicians.

To recap:

Do
- Know the definition of a PA and be able to articulate the major components
- Use the word collaboration when talking about the PA-Physician relationship
- Talk about your personal experiences with PAs

Don't
- Use mid-level provider or advance practice provider in your definition
- Use the work supervision to describe the PA-Physician relationship
- Say the dreaded Physician's Assistant

3. Why do you want to be a PA?

This is probably the most important question of your interview, as it gets to your motivations for pursuing a career in medicine and a career as a PA. Some applicants will have a singular moment that really guided them to want to be a PA or pursue a career in medicine, while others will not.

For either scenario, we provide a roadmap below for how to best answer this question.

In answering, you should start broad and then get more specific as you go. First, talk about why you want to be in medicine and healthcare. What interests you about it? What is exciting about it? What does the field offer to you that other fields simply do not? Here is also a time to talk about and he specific moment or moments that really drove you to pursue the medical field. Next, you should talk about your first exposure to the PA profession. How did you hear about it? Did you research it online or find out about it while working? What did you do to learn more about it? What was that first experience with a PA like? Finally, get into why you want to be a PA, and specifically, what you like about the job and role of a PA. Do you like the responsibility? Do you like the versatility? Do you like the different tasks that PAs are able to handle? Do you like the relationships that they have with other members of the health care team? How would being a PA provide you with daily joy and satisfaction?

Additionally, when entering this question there are some topics you should avoid. Firstly, there is a misconception that PAs generally have more time to spend with patients. In most situations that is not the case at all. In my primary care practice, I get the same amount of time with a patient as my physician colleagues. This is the case in most outpatient settings regardless of specialty. Another misconception is that PA have a better work-life balance. This is not necessarily true either. Your work-life balance is really what you make of it. You can choose to work only part time or per diem and have time for other important things in your life or you can work 80 hours a week, regardless of whether you are a PA or physician. In fact, PAs are sometimes hired to work the hours and do the tasks that the physician simply does not want to do. Finally, a common topic brought up is lateral mobility of PAs. It is true that we can work in any area of medicine and can transition to new areas during our career. However, it should not be your primary reason for choosing PA. Your primary reason should center around the role of the PA and working with patients.

Furthermore, this is not the time to bring up other professions if you can avoid it. You do not want to say, for example, that you are choosing to be a PA because it is less schooling than medical school. While this is true, it makes you seem like you are taking the easy way out or that you are not a hard worker and you don't want that to be the impression that the faculty member walks away from the interview with. There is also no need to bring up why you don't want to be a physician or a nurse practitioner or a physical therapist or any other profession at this time. However, you should still be prepared to answer that question if they follow up with that question.

To recap:

Do
- Talk about why medicine and healthcare in general
- Discuss your first exposure to PAs
- Discuss what you like about the role of PAs

Don't
- Use misconceptions (spending time with patients, work-life balance) as major reasons for wanting to be a PA
- Use lateral mobility as your primary reason for wanting to be a PA
- Bring up other professions (MD, DO, NP, etc)

4. Why do you want to be a PA opposed to a physician or nurse practitioner?

It is important in answering this question to show that you have researched these other professions to conclude that PA is what fits you best. You want to show that you are knowledgeable with professions and the role that they play on the healthcare team, while also having specific reasons for why PA is a better match for you.

There are several topics you could discuss when talking about why you want to be a PA versus a physician. Now is certainly a time where you can talk about lateral mobility and being able to work in different fields of medicine. You can also talk about the length of training that is required for physician as they typically do require four years of college, four years of medical school, and a minimum of three years of residency. If you are older or pursuing a second career you just may not have the desire to be in school for that long, and that is totally okay. Finally, you can also talk about personality traits that might be more in line with being a PA versus being a physician, or experiences that you have had with PAs or physicians that led you to pursue becoming a PA.

There are also several topics you could discuss in comparing the PA to the nurse practitioner. Firstly, nurse practitioners have to be registered nurses first before they can attend a nurse practitioner program. For many students it may not make sense to add this additional one to two years of training to their education to ultimately end up having a very similar role to a PA. Secondly, there are dramatic differences in their training. PAs are trained under the medical model, and are required to have approximately 2,000 hours of clinical rotations during their program. They are trained in general medicine. Nurse practitioners are trained under the nursing model. You should be able to describe how this is different from the medical model. Generally, their education is focused on one area (neonatology, psychiatry, primary care, acute care), and they complete fewer clinical hours during their education program. Finally, very few nurse practitioners first assist in surgery. If surgery is something you are interested in, it is dominated by PAs and would make more sense to go to PA school where you will have surgical training.

The most important thing in discussing the other professions is that you do not denigrate another profession. Everyone has an important role to play in patient care, and you want to show that you have respect and appreciation for the other professions and their roles. After all, these people will be your future coworkers and colleagues.

To recap:

Do
- Research and show your understanding of other health professions
- Articulate reasons for choosing PA over becoming a physician or nurse practitioner
- Discuss differences in training among the professions

Don't
- Denigrate another profession in your answer

5. Why do you want to come here for PA school?

In answering this question, you want to show the program that you are a good fit for their program. You need to relate your desires or life experiences to aspects of the program that resonate with you to show them that you are a good match for them.

In general, it is always a good idea to focus on the program mission statement. You can relate this mission statement to experiences in your life or to professional goals that you may have to show them that you are committed to fulfilling the program's mission. For example, if a program has a mission to serve the underserved, talk about any experiences you have in working with underserved populations. Additionally, you can focus on aspects of the curriculum that may resonate with you as well. Perhaps they have international rotations and one of your goals is to work abroad. Perhaps they have in addiction medicine elective and your primary interest is working in psychiatry. Show them that you have researched their curriculum and that there are specific reasons why their curriculum is a match for you. Finally, you can also discuss unique program features, clinical rotation sites, elective rotations, learning format, location, or any other aspect that made you apply to their program.

It is best to stay away from a few topics when talking about why you want to come to a particular school. There is generally no need to talk about PANCE pass rates. The vast majority of schools have rates that are over 90% and most of the ability to pass the certification exam comes down to the individual students and their studying rather than the program itself. All programs will teach you what you need to pass the PANCE. Even though attrition rates are now publicly available, I would also avoid talking about those. Most programs have very low attrition rates, and many times the students who do leave the program do so for non-academic reasons that the program could not have avoided. You want to show them that you are confident in your ability to complete the program, and student attrition can be a sore spot for many programs. Finally, it's best not to bring up specific statistics for acceptance into a program. You never want to say that you applied to a program because they have a slightly higher acceptance rate than another program or that it seemed easier to get into.

To recap:

Do
- Discuss the mission statement and how it resonates with you
- Talk about the curriculum and how it is a good fit for you and your goals
- Point out unique features of the program that make it a good fit for you

Don't
- Talk about PANCE pass rates
- Focus on student attrition
- Discuss admitted student statistics as a reason for why you applied

THE OTHER QUESTIONS

In this section, we will review some of the other common classic interview questions for PA programs. It would be impossible to review every single question that could be asked but many of the concepts from answering the questions that we will go over can be applied to other questions you may come across.

6. How has your academic work prepared you for PA school?

Here's your chance to tell the PA faculty why you are prepared to hit the ground running when you start PA school. They want you to show them that you can handle a rigorous academic workload. The biggest item to focus on here is time management. It is true that going to PA school is like trying to drink water out of a firehose. You want to show them that through your undergraduate career you have been able to manage your time among multiple priorities in order to be successful. You could perhaps highlight that you took multiple rigorous science classes at the same time and did well, or perhaps that you took a particularly heavy course load at 18 or 20 credits one semester and succeeded. If you are a non-traditional student or a traditional student with other responsibilities you could talk about managing your classwork with your other responsibilities including employment, family, clubs, extracurriculars, or athletics.

Similar Questions:
- What do you think will be challenging about PA school?
- What was your most challenging undergraduate course and why?
- How do you study?

7. Have you applied to other programs?

This is usually a very innocent question. Many programs are interested in learning what other programs are attracting their students and who they are competing with. Schools do not expect that you only will have applied to one program. They realize how hard it is to get into PA school. A simple answer would be to say that yes you have applied to several other programs. It is very difficult to get into PA school, and you wanted to give yourself the best chance of being accepted this cycle. You could also list the most important factors for you in choosing which programs you applied to such as curricular features, location, international opportunities or anything else you used to narrow down your list of programs. Finally, you can highlight that even though you applied to other programs, the program you're interviewing at is your top choice school and state why that is the case.

> ### Similar Questions:
> - Which other schools did you apply to?
> - How did you decide where to apply?
> - Why did you apply to our program?

8. Describe an interaction with a patient that made an impact on you.

This is a straightforward question. You should always have at least one or two patient experiences in your head to discuss during a PA school interview. The key here isn't so much the interaction that you had with the patient, but rather what did you learn from the interaction or what did you take away from the interaction that changed you in some meaningful way. In your answer, you should talk about the circumstances of the interaction such as where it occurred and when it occurred, while leaving out any privileged patient information. Describe what happened and what about it was impactful in your life. The impact could be that it changed your perspective, that you learned something new, or simply that it emboldened you to continue pursuing a career in medicine.

Similar Questions:
- What do you enjoy about working with patients?
- Tell me about a memorable patient experience
- How have you grown as a person from taking care of patients?

9. Describe a stressful situation you were in and how you dealt with it.

The faculty member wants to know if you will be able to handle the rigors of the academic program. Thus, here they are looking for insight as to what you find stressful and how you handle that stress. To answer this question, pick a stressful situation in your life. It could be an interpersonal, family, academic, or job-related situation. Tell the story of why that situation was particularly stressful, and then talk about how you were able to persevere. You could talk about various things that you do to relieve stress including exercise, going to church or religious services, prayer, yoga, meditation, spending time with pets, or anything else that is an outlet for you. The key is that you choose a situation that would be stress provoking for most people (i.e. not the time where you forgot to bring a pen to class), and that you had specific actions that you took to manage your stress successfully and achieve the desired outcome from the situation. You can then link it back to how you plan to use those tactics to handle stress while in PA school.

Similar Questions
- How do you deal with stress?
- What do you find stressful?
- What kind of stress do you seeing arising as a PA student or practicing PA?

10. What do you do outside of work or academics?

With this question, they are just trying to get to know you as a person more. This is the time to highlight any hobbies or interests that are not medically related that might help you to stand out from the crowd. They want to see that you are a well-rounded individual and not someone who has had their head in a book for the last four years during undergrad or were working 80 hour weeks and missing out on life. Some topics for discussion could include clubs, volunteering, travel, sports, music, family, writing, exercise, that half-marathon you just finished, or anything else that you have a genuine interest in and have dedicated time to. Generally, you should avoid topics related to money (i.e. gambling) or politics.

> ### Similar Questions:
> - What is your favorite hobby?
> - What do you like to do for fun?
> - What do you like to do in your spare time?

11. What are your strengths?

When answering this question, you want to tie back whatever strength or strengths you choose to how they will be helpful for you either as a PA student or as a practicing PA. It can be a difficult question to answer, as many applicants have a difficult time talking about themselves without feeling like they are bragging. This is your chance to brag! Try and think of the things that people compliment you on often. Some examples could be your time management, a personality trait, your ability to work with others, or your work ethic. You can even tell a story about how that strength has enabled you to be successful in your job, academics, or other arenas. Whichever strength or strengths you chose, make sure to link them back to how they will be helpful in PA school or as a PA.

- Why should we choose to accept you into our program?
- What is your best trait?
- What would your last or current boss say about you?

12. What are your weaknesses?

The aim of this question is to find out whether you are capable of self-reflection and working on improving yourself. There's something that everyone should be working on to better themselves. When answering this question, the first step is to state what your actual weakness is. Some common weaknesses that people will describe are being too passive, being a perfectionist, overcommitment, or a personality trait. Then you need to describe why you see this as a weakness, and what you are doing about it to turn it into a strength. If you have a story that exemplifies this, now is the time to tell it. For example, if your weakness is being a perfectionist, you can site examples of how you are learning to accept imperfection (whether it be in a class at school or after you make a mistake at work) and attempting to learn from the imperfections rather than let them define you as a person.

Similar Questions:
- What do people often criticize about you?
- What is one area of your life you are trying to improve upon?
- If you could change one thing about yourself, what would it be?

13. What will you do if you are not accepted to PA school this year?

In this answer, faculty are primarily looking to see that you are committed to pursuing the PA path. You want to have a thoughtful answer that shows that you have thought about the possibility of not being accepted, because it does take most students more than one cycle to be accepted. A good answer would be to discuss plans that you have to further improve your application including taking coursework, volunteering, shadowing, retaking standardized tests, and obtaining more patient care experience hours. You can even discuss reaching out to programs that you are not accepted at to see what they perceive your weaknesses to be and how you can improve upon those prior to the next cycle.

Alternatively, you want to avoid saying that you have applied to other health professions or that if you don't get into PA school your plan is to pursue a different career path. Even if this may be the case, it certainly is not what faculty would want to hear. They want to know that you are committed to PA, first and foremost. Additionally, if you have already been accepted to another PA program, you can let them know that fact, and follow up that statement with "however, this is my top choice program and that is why I chose to still interview here".

Similar Questions:
- What would you do if not accepted to our PA school this application cycle?
- What are your plans for the next year?
- What are some areas of your application you could improve upon?

14. Do you have any questions about our program?

This seemingly innocuous question is an important one. It certainly would be easy to say that you don't have any further questions and that all of your questions have been answered during the interview. However, it is better to have a few questions prepared in advance that you can ask during the interview as conversation starters. It shows the faculty that you are more interested in pursuing their program and that you have been very thoughtful in preparing for your interview. You should make sure that any questions you ask cannot simply be answered on their website or were not previously reviewed in other parts of the interview. Some common questions could include questions about the clinical rotation sites, extracurricular opportunities, leadership opportunities, or any opportunities to engage in research. For many programs, this information is not readily available on their website.

Similar Questions:
- Do you feel that you have a solid understanding of our program and what we offer?
- Are there any questions that we have not answered yet?
- Is there anything else you were hoping to discuss?

15. What did you gain from your healthcare experience?

To answer this question, it is important to do some self-reflection. Everyone will have different things that they take away from their healthcare experience. For some it might be simply learning how to interact with patients in members of the health care team, especially if it was your first job. For others you may have learned more about health care in the US health care system, both its strengths and its weaknesses. You may have become more adept at handling stressful situations such as injury or death. You may have grown as a person in other ways because of your interactions with patients. The key here is really to have thought about this before the interview and try and link it back to how your healthcare experience has made you a better person and prepared you for a career as a future PA. If you can articulate that, you will have a great answer ready to go.

Similar Questions:
- How did your healthcare experience prepare you for becoming a PA?
- What did you learn about yourself while working with patients?
- Why was your healthcare experience valuable?

16. What would be your ideal job?

There is some debate as to how to best answer this question. there are two reasonable approaches. The first approach would be to look at the mission statement of the program and describe a job that would be aligned with that program mission statement. for example, many PA programs have a focus on primary care, so if that is a genuine interest of yours you can talk about how you would ideally like to work in a primary care role in a community of your choosing. Other PA programs have different focuses such as a Pediatrics focus or a surgical focus and if those are interests of yours you can tailor your response to that as well. The second approach is to describe an ideal job based upon your previous experiences. For example, if you are a dermatology medical assistant, you could discuss how you want to be a dermatology PA. However, you should always leave the door open to other possibilities and show an open mind toward pursuing different specialties that you have not experienced yet in your career. You may fall in love with something else during clinical rotations.

Another important aspect to this question is that many PA programs are looking for someone who is going to do more than just clinical work. For example, they want to see that their graduates go on to pursue leadership roles, get involved in state or national organizations, do medical mission trips, precept PA students, teach in PA programs, or do anything else that can help to advance the profession. Thus, if you have similar aspirations, now is a great time to mention them and impress the faculty.

Similar Questions:
- After you graduate, what field do you plan to work in?
- Where do you see yourself in 5 years?
- How do you plan to contribute to the PA profession in the future?

17. What has been your biggest success?

This is a great chance to get to tell the interviewer something about your life that has meaning. Your biggest success could perhaps be something medically related to PA school, but it does not have to be. For those who have kids or who are married, these will typically be on the list of your biggest successes or achievements. For those who have overcome a seemingly insurmountable obstacle in their life, you may want to discuss that here. Perhaps you started a business in a former life, were a college or professional athlete, or completed a medical mission trip that was meaningful to you. This one takes some reflection, but in doing so you will be able to come up with a great answer and story that you might be able to use for other interview questions as well.

Similar Questions:
- What has been your greatest achievement?
- What is the best thing that has happened to you in your life?
- What are you the proudest of?

18. What has been your biggest failure?

This is a tough yet very important question. The faculty members want to see that you have reflected on mistakes in your life and have learned something from them. They also want to get an idea of what exactly you consider to be a failure, and it should be something major. Getting a bad grade on an exam in undergrad will not be the answer that they are looking for, so you will have to dig deep and really think this question through before your interview. You do not want to say that you have never experienced a major failure, as this is a red flag that you are not reflective or have not had the "life experience" needed to be successful in PA school. The failure can be a personal failure (perhaps relating to a relationship), an academic failure (perhaps you were put on probation or kicked out of school), or a professional failure (related to a current or former job). The key is that you describe the situation, what went wrong, and what you learned from it.

Similar Questions:
- What has been a major disappointment in your life?
- What is the worst thing that has happened to you in your life?
- What is your biggest life regret?

19. What do you know about the history of PAs?

As with any career, you want to have an understanding of the history of the career that you are pursuing. The PA profession is a fairly new profession having been around for only approximately 60 years. Though you don't need to know every single detail of the 60-year history of the profession you should have a general idea of the roots of the PA profession. In the 1960s there were a shortage of medical providers, primarily primary care providers in the United States. One of the ways to address this provider shortage was to come up with a new profession called the physician assistant, who was trained similar to a military medic under the medical school model. In fact, the first PAs were former Navy Corpsmen. The first PA program in the 1960s was at Duke University and was founded by Eugene Stead. Since then, PAs have gradually attained more autonomy and responsibilities and their influence in the medical system has increased drastically. There are now over 280 accredited PA programs and over 160,000 certified PAs in the United States.

Similar Questions:
- How did the PA profession come to be?
- Who is Eugene Stead?
- How long have PAs been around?

20. Who is the most important member of the healthcare team?

This is actually a fairly easy question, but one that definitely trips up applicants. When we think about the health care team of course we think about doctors, PAs, nurses, therapists, speech language pathologists and nursing assistants all as being a part of the team. However, the most important member of the health care team by far is the patient themself. After all, we are here to care for patients. The patient needs to feel as though they are a part of the team and that you are making decisions with them and with their input rather than on their behalf. The patient's biopsychosocial factors need to be considered in making care decisions and the only way to do that is to truly get to know them and involve them in their care. The only other reasonable way to answer this question is to state that there is no one singular more important role than another on the health care team. Everyone is vital to ensuring a good outcome for the patient, otherwise there would be no need for that person on the team. Overall, I think it's a safer bet to always put the patient first as the leader of the team, but you could probably get away with the alternative reply as well if you felt strongly about it.

Similar Questions:
- What role on the healthcare team is most important?
- Describe what patient-centered care means.
- Tell me about the biopsychosocial model of care.

21. What do you expect a typical day to be like for a PA student?

The most important thing in answering this question is to show that you have an understanding of how rigorous PA school actually is. It is not uncommon to have a few students in each class dropped out of the PA program within the first few weeks, just because their expectations for the workload were not on par with reality. When this happens, programs are often unable to fill those seats as the semester has already started and then they are left with open spots and no recourse. Hence, they like to ask this question to try and avoid that situation.

You should talk about the fact that in most programs you'll be in class for six to 8 hours a day five days a week and that after class you'll need to spend most of your time in the evening studying. You will have to make many sacrifices with family, friends, and other loved ones who you may not be able to see or interact with as much while in school. That's not to say that you shouldn't find time to do something fun every once in a while, or just take some time for yourself every week, but overall your life will largely be dominated by school and school work. During the clinical phase, your hours can vary from a typical eight to five day on an outpatient rotation to 80 hour works weeks on inpatient or surgical rotations. Then, after clinicals you will still need to study. It will be a balancing act between PA school and other life responsibilities, but in general most of your time will be dedicated to becoming the best provider that you can be.

Similar Questions:
- What daily routine do you envision while in PA school?
- Are you mentally prepared for the rigors of a PA program?
- Tell me about your expectations for studying during the PA program

22. What are your biggest support systems?

PA school is hard. There is no doubt that you will have times where you feel like giving up while in school. Thus, programs like to know that you have a strong support system that you can rely on during challenging times to help you succeed while in school. Your support system could be a spouse, other family members, friends who have completed the program previously or who are local to the area that the program is in, a church or other religious community, or any other organization or group that you are a part of that gives you guidance and strength. Talk about anyone who is supportive of your PA goals.

Similar Questions:
- How will you survive PA school?
- Who do you have to rely upon for support when times get challenging?
- Who has encouraged you to become a PA?

23. What was your hardest undergraduate class and why?

The class that you pick to answer this question really does not matter. What's most important is what you were able to learn about yourself or take away from the situation that might help you in PA school. For a lot of people, they may struggle with organic chemistry or general chemistry, yet other people struggle with math or perhaps a hard biology course. Tell them about your experience in this course and what you ultimately were able to do to be successful. Perhaps you developed better study skills or time management skills that will be useful for you in PA school. Perhaps you were going through a difficult time in another aspect of your life, and that made the class more challenging than it needed to be. Wrap up by showing how you overcame whatever obstacle there was, and how now you are more ready for PA school than ever because of that experience.

Similar Questions:
- Tell me about a difficult class you had in undergrad
- Tell me about your most challenging class and how you were able to succeed
- What did you learn about yourself during your hardest undergraduate class?

24. What do you think is the biggest challenge facing PAs?

There are many challenges that are facing PAs today. One challenge that comes to mind is increasing autonomy of PAs under what is called optimal team practice. This essentially means allowing PAs to provide care to the highest level that their training allows them to do. Nurse practitioners have been very successful in advocating for independent practice in many states, and now PAs are trying to do the same to expand access to care and remain on a level playing field with nurse practitioners. Another challenge that you could discuss would be the public perception of PAs. Many patients really do not have a good understanding of the role and responsibilities of the PA, their education and training, and their ability to provide quality care to patients. Even within the medical team, there are often members who fully do not understand the role of the PA. It is our job and responsibilities to improve that understanding. We encourage you to research these and other challenges, and have a general understanding of the issues that PAs face prior to your interview.

Similar Questions
- What challenges do you see ahead in practicing as a PA?
- What negatives are there about being a PA?
- What do you plan to do to help tackle some of the issues that the PA profession faces?

25. What are your thoughts on the name change from physician assistant to physician associate?

This is an interesting question and it is important to know the background. The first PA programs were actually physician associate programs. In fact, two programs currently are still called physician associate programs at Yale University and the University of Oklahoma. Over time, the title was transitioned to physician assistant as it was felt that this was a more appropriate name in the infancy of the profession. More recently, as PAs have expanded their roles and responsibility, there has been a name change debate. Many PAs feel as though the title physician assistant is confusing as we really do not assist physicians and it can very easily be confused for medical assistant for example. Because of this, the American Academy of PAs invested $1 million into a market research project to determine what the best name for the profession would be. Market research found that the best name for the profession would be medical care practitioner. However, the House of delegates at the American Academy of PAs national meeting voted to change the name to physician associate. This was the original name of the profession, and this would not require us to change our initials. As you can imagine, there is some controversy around this subject.

Most PAs at least feel that physician associate is better than physician assistant, as it better describes who we are. Interestingly, physician associate is also the terminology used for our profession in Canada and Great Britain as well. Most PAs think that by changing the name, it will be easier to move onward with legislative agendas and get more laws favoring PAs. The major cons to the name change are that it could be confusing to patients, and that we ultimately did not decide on the name that was supported by the research, physicians, and other stakeholders.

CHAPTER 3: SITUATIONAL INTERVIEW QUESTIONS

INTRODUCTION:

Situational questions, also known as behavioral questions, generally require you to think back to and describe a situation from your life. Usually, the topics are similar to the traditional style questions, but you use examples to illustrate your message in your answers. For example, an interviewer could ask you "how do you deal with conflict?". This would be a more classic question. However, they could also ask, "Describe a situation where there was conflict and how it was resolved". Here, they are trying to get you to recall a situation in your life where you displayed a desired behavior (conflict resolution). As you can imagine, the themes of your answer will be the same. However, your answer itself will be different depending on how it is phrased.

When describing a situation there are a few things to keep in mind. Firstly, make sure to give adequate background information so that your interviewer can understand the story you tell. Secondly, point out how the story is relevant to the question you were asked, if it is not obvious. Thirdly, talk about how the situation was resolved, and what you learned from it. Finally, if possible, try to relate this back to being in PA school or being a PA and how it might help you. For example, you could say that from the situation you learned about to be an effective mediator. You could then talk about how these skills could be useful as a PA when you are working with a patient and family members who may not agree on a treatment plan or course of action.

Lastly, and most importantly, in any situation or scenario that involves a patient, remember to always put the patient first. In doing so, you will almost always arise at an acceptable answer for the given question.

We have attempted to cover the most commonly asked situational questions and themes, though of course it would be impossible to cover them all. We definitely recommend searching the web, forums, and other resources to get additional practice.

QUESTIONS:

1. Describe what you would do if your collaborating physician told you to do something that you thought was wrong for a patient.

This is a very common question that is asked during interviews. It is both a behavioral question as well as an ethical question. This question aims at determining whether you understand the role of the PA as well as the relationship between the PA and the collaborating physician. The key here is that in any situation you always need to put the safety and care of the patient above all else.

In your answer you should aim to have a conversation with your collaborating physician and discuss any concerns that you may have about their request. Perhaps you're not quite understanding the request or there's something that you are missing about the patient's history which may pertain to the decision being made by your physician. It is also entirely possible that the physician is making a mistake that they don't realize, as no one is perfect. Ultimately, your interviewer needs to see that you will stand up for your patient, and that you will handle the situation professionally. The wrong answer would be to say that you will simply follow whatever the collaborating physician tells you to do, regardless of whether you feel comfortable with it or not.

2. Have you ever seen someone die?

In this question the interviewer is trying to get a better understanding of your life experience. If you have seen someone die in front of you, this is the opportunity to describe the situation and reflect upon that experience and what you took away from it. You can also link this to how you might act in a similar situation if you are a health care provider and a patient passes away in front of you and other family members. It would be a good time to discuss empathy and compassion.

If you have not ever seen someone die in front of you, that is okay. You can simply state that you have not, but then also try and discuss the passing of a family member or friend that had an impact on you. Talk about what you took away from that situation that has changed you as a person and what you learned from it that you can apply in your life and as a future PA.

3. What would you do if you saw a classmate cheating on an exam?

This is a classic ethical and behavioral question. It is also a very straightforward question to answer. If you have any suspicions that a classmate is cheating, your best bet is always to bring this to the attention of faculty members so that it can be handled appropriately. If a classmate is truly cheating, that clearly raises concerns about their ethics and their ability to provide ethical care as a health care provider in the future and it would need to be addressed by the program. If you had a good relationship with that student, you could also directly discuss your concerns with them, though this could lead to further conflict so it is best to tread lightly. If you have experienced this in your undergraduate career, you could also discuss how you handled it and how it was resolved.

The wrong answer would be to simply do nothing or turn a blind eye to a potential problem. As a future healthcare provider, it is important to be able to speak up when you see something that is wrong. Additionally, it is important to recognize that this person who is cheating could become a future health care provider that may engage in unethical conduct with patients, whom could be your family members or friends. It is better to address it now, then have a future patient be affected.

4. Describe how you would handle an interaction with a difficult patient.

Anyone who has worked in healthcare in any capacity has had patients that are difficult to work with. This could be because of their diagnosis, personality conflicts, family dynamics or other reasons. The key to answering this question is to choose an interaction you've had with a difficult patient, describe why it was difficult, discuss how you were able to overcome those difficulties, and to discuss what you learned from this encounter that you can use in future patient encounters.

The wrong way to answer this question would be to say that you've never had a difficult patient encounter. For one, this just simply isn't believable if you've been working in healthcare. Secondly, if you've really never had a difficult patient, that reveals a lack of experience in the medical field that you would not want to highlight during your interview. The word "difficult" can mean different things to different people, so anyone should really be able to come up with a situation that was "difficult" to discuss.

5. Tell me about a time when you needed to ask for help.

One of the most important concepts in medicine and as a PA is knowing when to ask colleagues for help (in medicine we call it "knowing what you don't know"). It shows that you are self-aware of your knowledge and skills, and that if something is beyond your abilities or expertise you will respond appropriately by asking for assistance or referring the patient to someone who is better able to help them.

In this question, the interviewer wants you to show your self-awareness that you are indeed not perfect and know when you are in over your head and need help. This could be related to academics, social life, personal life, family life, or any other area. It does not have to be related to your job or medicine. Describe the situation, why you needed to ask for help, and what the outcome ultimately was. Show that you were self-aware, willing to work with someone else (perhaps as a team) to solve a problem, and what you learned from the situation.

The wrong answer would be stating that you never have needed to ask someone for help. This would come across as narcissistic and would make you seem like someone who does not work well with others.

6. What would you do if someone in your class was suffering from a drug or alcohol problem?

PA school is very stressful and it is possible for students to handle stress inappropriately by turning to drugs or alcohol. If you suspect that a classmate is suffering from a drug or alcohol problem, your goal should be to get them help. You could discuss your concerns with them openly and honestly, try to link them to community resources that may be of assistance, and also engage them with faculty members that may be able to assist them as well.

The wrong answer would be to do nothing. Not only could this have devastating consequences for them as a person, but it could also lead to endangerment of patients in the future. You also want to be non-judgmental. You do not want to make them feel bad for their decisions.

7. Tell us about a time when you demonstrated compassion.

To answer this question, your best bet is to refer back to an interaction that you had with a patient where you demonstrated compassion. It does not need to be something extravagant, such as comforting the family members of a patient who recently passed away. It can be something simple like helping a COVID patient learn to use an iPad so that they are able to FaceTime with family members and friends while they're in the hospital, or grabbing them their favorite magazine to read from the gift shop. Sometimes it is the littlest things that can make the biggest difference for a patient, and it is important to show that you understand that concept.

Another option would be to discuss a situation from your personal life where you showed compassion to a family member or friend. The theme of the answer would be the same, but the context would be different. If your best example of showing compassion is outside the realm of medicine, that is totally okay and you should use that as your answer. Overall, make sure to show that you understand what compassion is and that you are a compassionate person.

8. Describe a situation where you were criticized and what your reaction was to the criticism.

Everyone has been criticized at some point in their life. The purpose of this question is to gauge how you respond to criticism. Feedback and criticism are essential to helping you grow as a person and as a healthcare provider. Thus, it is important to not react to it negatively, but rather try and learn something from the situation that you can improve on in the future. Examples could come from school, the workplace, or interactions with friends or family members. Show that you can be introspective.

The wrong answer would be to say either that you have never been criticized or that when you are criticized you tend not to take it to heart and just ignore the feedback. Even when criticism is not constructive, there are always lessons that can be learned.

9. What is the biggest challenge you have overcome in your life?

There are two purposes to this question. The first purpose is to understand what types of things you actually find challenging. The second purpose is to see what strategies you use to overcome challenges in your life. The challenge you choose to describe can be a personal, academic, professional challenge. Perhaps you have been overweight for most of your life and you can describe your weight loss journey. Perhaps you were faced with a difficult situation in the workplace that you had to overcome. The key here is to choose something in your life that was challenging and meaningful to you and to describe healthy strategies and habits that you used to overcome that challenge. Show your work ethic, initiative, creative thinking, or other personal attributes that helped you persevere. End your answer by discussing what you learned from that situation and how you can apply it to other aspects of your life or to becoming a PA.

The wrong answer would of course be to say that you haven't experienced any large challenges in your life. PA schools are generally looking for mature students who have life experience that they can bring to the classroom and program. You want to show that you that you have faced some adversity and been able to overcome it.

10. Tell us about a time where you showed initiative.

The key to answering this question is showing that you can take a difficult situation in your own hands and come up with a solution to solve a problem. It does not have to be overly complicated.

For example, when I was in PA school I wanted to complete a medical education elective. However, this elective was only offered to medical students and there had never been a PA student who had completed the course. I took the initiative to set up a meeting between the course director and a faculty member in my program. In this meeting we were able to discuss how this course would be of benefit for me and foster interprofessional collaboration between the PA program and the medical students. Ultimately, I was able to complete the elective and subsequently several other PA students have as well.

Choose a situation where you took initiative to solve a problem in your workplace or academic career. Describe the circumstances and how you came up with and enacted a solution. End your answer by stating that it can be difficult for change to take place, but that with persistence you can make a meaningful difference.

11. Say you are a PA and your patient is terminally ill. The patient looks at you, with hope, and asks if he will make it. What do you tell them?

This is a challenging question. The most important thing to remember is that you need to be honest with your patient. Communicating bad news is never easy. You want to be as empathetic as possible. You can certainly tell them that their chances are slim, and try to give them your best estimate for how much time they may have left so they can spend their remaining days doing the things they love and enjoy most. Try to end with a message of hope for things that they will be able to do in the future, no matter how long that future may be (see family and friends, go on a trip, etc).

The wrong answer would be to lie and tell them that their chances are great for a full recovery. It might be easiest to say this in the moment, but as PAs we need to be comfortable having difficult conversations with our patients. They'll appreciate you more for being honest.

12. Imagine you are a PA and working with a patient who refuses a treatment that you think is necessary. What would you do?

Ultimately the patient has the right to refuse treatment for any condition. In answering this question, you want to emphasize that you will do your best to educate the patient. Tell them about the benefits of the treatment but also tell them about the potential risks of the treatment. Talked to them in a straightforward way about why you think this treatment is the best course of action for them and also listen to their concerns and do the best you can to assuage those fears. Many times patients are simply afraid of the unknown and by taking a little bit of extra time to discuss their concerns, you can convince them on treatment.

The wrong answer would be to simply "give up" on the patient or get frustrated or angry at them. We have to realize that patient's come in with their own perspective and life experiences that affect their decision making. All we can do as providers is educate them and offer our best advice.

13. Describe a disappointing moment in your life and what you learned from it.

Everyone has been disappointed by something in their life. However, in answering this question, the disappointing moment isn't all that important. Rather, what is important is how you reacted and what you learned from the experience. The moment does not have to be a particularly significant situation. Examples could include academics, athletics, personal life, or others. Many students utilize this opportunity to address a course they may not have done well in or even the fact that they did not get accepted into PA school the first time that they applied. This is a great opportunity to show how you react to unexpected outcomes, how you have grown as a person, and what steps you have taken to improve yourself.

The only way you can go wrong with this question is to state that you've never had a disappointing moment in your life. Always do your best to provide an example, no matter how big or small.

14. Describe a time that you have struggled academically and how you dealt with it.

Almost everyone has struggled at some point during their academic career whether it be in a particular course or during a semester or perhaps simply due to immaturity. It is likely that you are going to struggle at some point in PA school simply because of the volume of information and the speed with which it comes at you. Faculty members want to know that you are resilient, resourceful, and are willing to put in the extra work or seek out additional help when needed. Describe an example where you were struggling. Discuss the steps that you took to remedy the situation and the ultimate outcome.

If you are the rare student who has no blemishes on their academic record, discuss what your plan would be if you are struggling in PA school. Would you adjust your study strategies? Would you reach out to faculty members for help? Would you group study with classmates? Let them know that even though you did well during undergraduate studies, you are aware how difficult PA school will be and will use any resources available to be successful. The only way you can go wrong with this question is to say that you never struggled during undergraduate and don't see yourself struggling at all in PA school.

15. How would you deal with a patient who refuses to see a PA and wants to only see a physician?

This situation does arise occasionally in clinical practice. It's an important situation to get comfortable with, and it is important not to become defensive or offended if the patient asks to see a physician or even simply another provider in the practice. Many patients do not fully understand what a PA is and sometimes a little education can go a long way.

If presented with this scenario do your best to introduce yourself, explain your role and your education. Also, explain to the patient that you would be happy to have them see the physician, but that they may need to reschedule if the physician is not available right now. Ultimately, they do get to pick who they see. Always keep things professional and remain composed. If they do agree to see you, use it as an opportunity to provide them with high quality care and represent the profession well so that in the future they will be happy to see PAs.

16. Tell us about your favorite team that you have been on.

Teamwork is important in healthcare and being a member of the health care team is what being a PA is all about. Faculty members want to know that you can be a team player and work with various other medical professionals. To answer this question, pick a team that you have been on in the past. This could be a sports team, work team, a lab group in college, or any other team you were part of. You could talk about a problem or challenge that you were able to overcome together and how you did that. You can also talk about what was so great about being on that team and what characteristics of that team made it successful. Always try to link this back to how you will be a team player as a future PA.

17. A patient attempts to contact you through social media. What would you do?

With this question, the interviewer is trying to see if you understand appropriate interactions between patients and health care providers. In nearly any circumstance, it is inappropriate to contact patients through social media. It is important to keep a professional relationship with your patients, and becoming "friends" with them on social media or otherwise, violates that relationship and can lead to conflicts of interest in the future. Conversely, if you have a great friend who wants to become a patient of yours, the same principles would apply. In general, you can be one or the other, but not both.

18. Tell me about a time where you showed professionalism.

To answer this question, you have to have a solid understanding of what professionalism means to you. There is a general definition of professionalism, but it certainly varies a bit from person to person. Before answering, think about what professionalism means to you and define that to your interviewer. Then, talk about a situation where you exhibited the characteristics of your definition of professionalism. Most of the time, examples will come from a workplace setting.

For example, if your definition of professionalism includes respect, kindness, confidence, and humility, you should discuss a situation in the workplace where you displayed those traits. It can be something simple. Don't overthink this one.

19. What would you do if your PA colleague came to work drunk?

There are two important parts of this question. The first is patient safety and the second is getting help for your colleague. In order to keep patients safe, it would be best to cancel any appointments that this colleague had scheduled with patients for the day. Once this is done, you could then discuss with your colleague what exactly happened. Perhaps they simply forgot that they had work that day and drank a little bit too much the night before but did not want to call out. Perhaps they truly have a problem with alcohol, and if that is the case you could certainly direct them to resources that might be helpful. It would also be important to report this situation to human resources so that they could intervene in an appropriate way.

The wrong answer would be to do nothing and allow your colleague to see patients. This would compromise patient safety.

20. Describe a time where you had to deal with conflict at work.

In every work setting, there can be conflict. It may be a simple conflict between two coworkers or something more complicated. The key to answering this question is to show that you've experienced conflict at work and that you were able to keep your composure and respond to conflict in a professional manner that led to a resolution of the conflict. Do not make things personal, and always try to understand the alternative perspective. Do your best to compromise (as long as it is not patient safety related) with the other person. The example you use can be as simple as a work scheduling conflict (who gets what holidays off).

CHAPTER 4: ETHICAL INTERVIEW QUESTIONS

INTRODUCTION:

Ethical interview questions or dilemmas are a common type of PA school interview question, and also can be a stumbling block for prospective students who have not prepared for these questions or experienced similar situations during their prior healthcare experience. Most commonly, the provided scenarios involve something related to a patient and/or their family. However, questions could also be completely unrelated to medicine at all. Here are a few pointers to help you think through how to answer these questions:

One of the major reasons these questions are asked is to uncover the moral standards of the interviewee and see if they match those of the institution. Thus, the first tip is to emphasize the importance of ethics and morals in your decision-making process. It is essential to include reasons why ethics are important in every answer given and to avoid saying that you have never experienced an ethical dilemma. We all have had our moral standards challenged at some point, so it is important to convey both the situations and how it was handled to the interviewer in the most compelling way possible. Additionally, be sure to relate how the ethical qualities you conveyed in your answer are important to medicine and patient care.

The second tip is to come prepared with an ethical dilemma you have faced in your life. Sometimes, rather than providing a scenario, you will simply be asked to describe an ethical/moral dilemma you have faced. Isolate a specific instance in which your ethics were challenged and be able to explain the situation, your task, your actions taken, and the end result. In general, this is a good format to follow for answering these types of questions, even when faced with a specific scenario during the interview. Our final tip is that for any ethical situation, you should try to acknowledge both points of view. This shows that you have thought through the situation thoroughly, and taken into consideration all sides of the scenario. However, be sure to decisively choose one point of view that you support and explain why you chose that path. This is another way for you to showcase your problem solving abilities and decision-making skills If there are any legal issues involved in the decision, be sure to address those as well.

Additionally, you should familiarize yourself with several important medical ethics concepts. These include:

1   Autonomy
2   Beneficience
3   Nonmalficience
4   Justice

A patient has autonomy when they are primarily responsible for their medical treatment plans. The provider may educate or advise the patient, but in the end, they must respect the patient's right to drive the decision, in other words, exercise autonomy.

A provider exhibits beneficence when they act solely with the patient's best interest in mind. All treatments benefit the patient, and the benefits outweigh the harms. Nonmaleficence states that a physician should do no harm to patients. Providers apply this principle when deciding between a medical intervention and doing nothing.

Finally, there is the concept of justice. This refers to whether a particular medical intervention is good for society and whether or not it violates any laws.

We have attempted to cover the most commonly asked ethical questions and themes, though of course it would be impossible to cover them all. We definitely recommend searching the web, forums, and other resources to get additional practice.

QUESTIONS:

1. Tell us about a medical ethics issue that you are passionate about.

This is an open-ended question, which is great because you get to pick a topic that you are knowledgeable about. There are several "hot button" topics right now that might be relevant. Some ideas for topics to discuss include:

- Healthcare reform
- Epidemic of drugs of abuse
- Physician-assisted suicide
- Access to abortion
- Socialized medicine
- Legalizing marijuana

Ultimately, your best bet here is to pick a topic you are knowledgeable about, and start by stating the context of the controversy. Discuss the two sides of the issue, and state your case for which side you believe is right and why. Try to avoid anything political in your response and always remember to put the patient first. You won't be penalized if your thoughts don't align with that of your interviewer, as long as you show critical thinking and that you consider and understand both sides of the argument.

Similar Questions
- What do you think is the most important issue in healthcare currently, and why?
- Have you ever had to make an ethical decision?
- What are your thoughts on treating family members or friends for their medical ailments?

2. You encounter a patient with HIV, and they do not want to tell their sexual partners. How would you respond?

Patients with HIV have the same rights to privacy as any other patient, and should always be treated in a non-judgmental fashion. Though there is a lot of stigma surrounding the disease and diagnosis, educating yourself about it can go a long way to alleviate any fears or biases you might have.

It is important to have a conversation with the patient to dispel any misinformation they may have regarding the diagnosis and ease any fears they may have. It is also important to discuss with them that it is imperative their partners be informed so that they can be treated and that the spread can be prevented even further. Don't place any blame on the patient for contracting this disease. After all, they got it from someone who may not have known or told them that they were infected. This is where developing a good relationship with a patient can make all the difference.

Many states have laws regarding this topic, and as a PA, you may be required to report a positive test to state or local health departments. If you are not sure what the laws are in your state, look them up! If you don't look them up before the interview, it is totally okay to state that you would have to look into what the law requires in your particular state as far as mandated reporting.

Here is a great resource where you can read more about this important issue: CDC website titled "HIV and STD Criminalization Laws".

Similar Questions:
- Would you still be willing to treat a patient who has HIV or AIDS? Why or why not?
- What would you do if you diagnose a patient with gonorrhea, but they do not plan to tell their sexual partners?

3. You are a PA and a physician colleague asks you to do something that you believe is wrong in caring for a patient. What do you do?

The key to answering this question is that you must always put the patient first. If you believe that a course of action recommended by a physician is wrong or harmful, you should not do it just because your collaborating physician asks you to. Ultimately, you have autonomy as a provider to do only what you feel is best and what you are comfortable with.

Do some research on the patient. Review their chart and speak with other members of the healthcare team to get a better picture of exactly what is going on, and then reach out to your collaborating physician.

You should have a conversation with your supervising physician and state your concerns. Perhaps there was something about the patient that you didn't know about that would make the physician's plan of care correct? Maybe they made a mistake, and after a collegial discussion they might agree with what you think is best. It could even be something as simple as them confusing two patients that might be in the office at the same time! Never rush to judgement. Stand up for what you think is right, but don't jump to blame or chastise your colleague who may have just made an honest mistake.

Ultimately, every provider has the same goal in mind, which is to do what is best for the patient. We all recite similar oaths in school, to do no harm and do all that we can to advocate for our patient and their health. Keep this in mind in a situation like this where there may be a disagreement.

Similar Questions:
- Your physician colleagues asks you to perform a procedure on a patient that you have never done before. What would you do?
- You are a patient's primary care PA and you receive a cardiologist's office notes for your patient. You disagree with the specialist's recommendations for treatment of their heart failure. What would you do?

4. You work as a primary care PA and you get samples of medications from pharmaceutical representatives to give to patients. While at work, you see a nurse taking a medication and bringing it to her car. What would you do?

Taking any medication without authorization from a prescriber is obviously inappropriate. Not only are these samples not meant for them, but they could be potentially harmful to your staff member if taken without a review of their other medications, medical history, etc. It also raises a red flag that this person may be unethical, stealing other things in the office, or have a substance abuse issue depending on what medications were taken.

It is your responsibility to take action as someone who witnessed this act. Doing nothing is not an option, as your ethics would not be looked upon favorably if someone found out that you knew about the issue and failed to act.

One reasonable solution would be to report this issue to your supervisor, human resources or practice management. They can then speak to the employee and take whatever action they deem to be appropriate. You could certainly, out of concern for the safety and wellbeing of the nurse, approach the nurse about what you saw. Even if they have what amounts to an "innocent" explanation (perhaps they have a prescription for that medication but just haven't gotten to the pharmacy to pick it up yet), it still makes sense to report to your supervisor.

Similar Questions:
- You witness a colleague taking a patient's left over medication that they brought to the office for disposal. What would you do?
- What would you do if you saw a classmate clearly cheating on an exam or an assignment?

5. *Your collaborating physician comes to work one morning and appears intoxicated. They insist they are fine and plan to go see their patients for the day. What would you do?*

As with most ethical questions, this comes down to putting the patient first. You can not allow an impaired provider to see patients as it may put the patient in harms way. Whether you are a PA, PA student, medical assistant, or anyone else on the healthcare team, it is imperative that you act.

Options for dealing with this situation would include: (1) Talking to the physician and expressing your concerns. Perhaps they would agree that it's best they call out for the day and come back tomorrow; (2) Let a supervisor know if you do not feel comfortable speaking with them directly; (3) You could consider reporting this behavior to the medical board in your state or even contacting police if they absolutely refused to heed to your requests.

As long as you show that you would act in some reasonable way, your interviewer will be pleased with your response.

Similar Questions
- You suspect a colleague has a substance abuse issue. What would you do?

6. *A patient comes into the ER with chest pain. You do an initial workup and decide it would be best to admit the patient overnight for observation. The patient refuses and wants to leave against your advice. What do you do?*

In this scenario, assuming the patient is of sound mind, they have the right to leave against medical advice. It is your responsibility as a provider to discuss with them the risks of leaving, and why you want them to stay. You need to show them that you are concerned for their health and that something bad could happen if they leave without completed your recommended treatment plan. If you do not seem to be able to get through to the patient, you could have other team members talk with the patient as well before they leave to see if they can change their mind.

If they still decide to leave, encourage them to come back if their symptoms worsen in any way, and follow up as soon as possible with their primary care provider. You could even reach out to them the next day to see how they are doing.

You see a patient in the office for a urinary infection, and prescribe them an antibiotic that they are allergic to by mistake. What should you do?

Everyone makes mistakes, and a similar situation will no doubt arise when you are practicing as a PA. The key is to own up to the mistake, put the patient first, and make sure you do everything in your power to inform the patient and make sure that they are safe from harm.

You should immediately reach out to the patient and let them know of the error and make sure they do not take the medication. If they have already started the medication, advise them not to take more of it. If they are developing any signs of severe allergy or they are known to have severe allergy to the medication, they should call 911 and proceed to the ER. If you can not get in touch with the patient, you should leave them a message. You can also call the local police department to visit their house for a well check to make sure that they are okay.

Another idea is to also call the pharmacy, to see if the patient picked up the medication or not. If not, you can cancel the prescription and send in an alternative that they are not allergic to. Make sure to have the pharmacy document their allergy as well, so that if an error is made in the future, it would be caught at the pharmacy.

The only way to answer this wrong is to say that you would do nothing and hope for the best. This could put a patient in harms way, and of course our duty as providers is first and foremost to do no harm.

Similar Questions:
- You prescribe the wrong dose of a medication for a patient. What would you do?
- Your nurse mixed up patients and sent in the wrong medication for one of your patients. What would you do?
- Your patient calls in looking for results of their lab work or imaging, but you forgot to order it. How would you approach this?

7. What are your thoughts on abortion?

This is a hot button topic given the current state of politics in the United States. Regardless of whether you are pro-choice or pro-life, it is important that you need to put those political views aside to do what is best for the patient. During the interview, it is okay to state your opinion on the issue, but your opinion should not cloud your caring for the patient.

If a patient were to come to you asking for an abortion, you need to do what is best for the patient. Provide them with resources as to how to access abortion care. Always remain non-judgmental. If you do not feel comfortable caring for a patient with this request, refer them to a colleague who is comfortable or better equipped to care for their needs. Always offer to be their advocate, and be a supportive listener. These decisions are never easy for the patient.

Similar Questions:
- What are your thoughts on recent "right to die" bills?
- Would you ever prescribe a placebo treatment, simply because the patient wants some type of treatment?
- Would you ever withhold a diagnosis from a patient?

8. You are seeing a gunshot victim in the ER and they are losing blood rapidly. The patient adamantly refuses blood transfusions, even though they might be lifesaving. What do you do?

This is a common ethical scenario, as it is well known that Jehovah's Witnesses often decline blood transfusions. This question gets back to the concept of patient autonomy. Ultimately, the patient gets to make their own medical decisions. You can provide them the benefits and risks, and encourage them to do what you think is in their best health interests, but they get to make the final decision.

In this case, you should certainly let them know that you think it is in their best interest to get transfused, and that without a transfusion, they may not survive. If they still decline, you should continue to do all you can to save the patient, short of giving a blood transfusion. Try not to get frustrated when patients do not follow your advice, as it will happen often. Your job is to present them with the information they need to make an informed decision, and then based on their preferences, care for them in the best way that you can.

Similar Questions:
- You advise your patient with diabetes that it is time to start medication, as their blood sugar is dangerously high. They do not want to take medication and instead want to try to manage it on their own. What do you do?
- A patient of yours is losing weight and has blood in their stool. You advise them that they need a colonoscopy, but they refuse. What do you do?

9. You're treating a 14-year-old female patient. Although the patient is below the legal age of consent, they reveal to you that they are sexually active. Do you confront their parents?

In this scenario, there are two main factors to consider. On the one hand, the patient is potentially engaging in illegal underage activities that may put their safety at risk (sex as a minor). On the other hand, the patient trusts you with this information, and you don't want to break provider-patient confidentiality.

Beneficence means that, as a provider, you must promote the course of action you believe is in the patient's best interest. In this case, that would mean encouraging the underage patient to inform their legal guardians they're sexually active as long as they feel safe doing so.

The mental well-being of the young patient is at risk since the situation suggests the patient could be taken advantage of. As a provider, you can offer contraception and sexual health advice without notifying the legal guardians. However, at the same time, confidentiality can be breached if the patient's safety is at risk.

Ultimately, this is a judgment call. If the patient were to tell you her sexual partner was 20 years old, that would constitute rape and would absolutely be reportable to parents and/or law enforcement, as the health and well being of the child are threatened. Otherwise, if there are no signs of harm to the patient, and you feel that your patient has a good relationship with her parents, encouraging them to discuss with their parents and offering contraception and/or sexual health advice may be all that is called for.

Similar Questions:
- Your teenage patient reveals to you that they were physically abused as a young child, but it has not happened in many years. What would you do?

- Your teenage patient with history of severe depression reveals that there are several guns throughout the house that are unlocked, as their dad is a hunter. What would you do?

CHAPTER 5: THE MMI INTERVIEW

INTRODUCTION:

Multiple Mini Interviews (MMI) are short 5 to 10 minute interviews that can happen with faculty members, staff, alumni, or other community members. Most often they are scenario based and you will be given a scenario prior to entering each room that you either have to act out or respond to. Sometimes the interviewer will also ask follow-up questions, while other times they are intentionally mute and simply there to observe your behavior and responses. Usually, programs will have six to eight stations that students will cycle through. Topics can include ethical questions, patient scenarios, behavioral questions, critical thinking exercises, problem solving exercises, and others. Programs will sometimes use a station to get a writing sample as well.

WHY DO ADMISSIONS COMMITTEES USE THIS FORMAT?

Based on research, MMI interviews offer many benefits to the admissions committee. They create a more reliable assessment of a candidate's strength and weaknesses, and help to limit biases from faculty members by creating multiple interactions. They also allow an applicant several opportunities to showcase their strengths, personality, and skills.

Finally, they allow the candidate to meet and interact with multiple members of the PA Program faculty to get a better sense of "fit" for a particular program. Schools will often tailor their stations to address important aspects related to the program mission statement or goals. The stations can help the applicant determine what a school stands for and what they are looking for in their applicants.

PREPARING FOR THE MMI INTERVIEW:

The MMI interview does not assess specific knowledge. It would be impossible to practice and prepare for all the potential scenarios and questions that could be asked. Instead, it is important to practice expressing yourself in a logical fashion in a timed environment when confronted with a challenging question.

To start, make sure that you research the program extensively including the mission statement, goals, curriculum, and any program themes that resonate with you as an applicant. Next, use the internet to search for potential MMI style questions, and practice responding to them in a thoughtful manner. The goal here is not to memorize a response, but instead practice thinking through a challenging question and articulating a coherent response in a defined amount of time. Practice with a friend or family member who can help point out flaws in your responses or times when your answer or body language may be awkward so you can address these things prior to your interview.

Finally, do your best to maintain your composure. If you are not sure how to answer a question, talk through your thought process with the interviewer and take a few moments to gather your thoughts. Often times, schools are more interested in how you think about a scenario than they are the ultimate answer that you provide to the prompt.

SAMPLE MMI QUESTIONS:

Below is a list of sample MMI questions that you can practice with.

1. What would you do if a family member with cancer decided to treat it solely with alternative medicine rather than standard medical treatment?

2. Your mother calls you and asks you to help with a major family decision. Your maternal grandfather is 75 years old and has been diagnosed with a condition that will kill him some time in the next three years. He can have a procedure that will correct the disease and not leave him with any long-term problems, but the procedure has a 20% mortality rate. He wants to have the procedure, but your mother does not want him to. How would you help mediate this issue?

3. You are a geneticist. One of your patients, Mary, had a boy with a genetic defect that may have a high recurrence risk, meaning her subsequent pregnancies has a high chance of being affected by the same defect. You offered genetic testing of Mary and her family to find out more about their disease, to which everyone agreed. The result showed that neither Linda nor her husband carry the mutation, while the boy inherited the mutation on a paternal chromosome that did not come from Linda's husband. In other words, the boy's biological father is someone else, who is unaware that he carries the mutation. You suspect that Mary nor her husband are aware of this non-paternity. How would you disclose the results of this genetic analysis to Linda and her family?

4. A 25 year old female patient of yours with Down's Syndrome becomes pregnant. The patient wants to keep the pregnancy but her mother and father want her to have an abortion and they come to your office for advice. How would you handle this situation?

5. Your PA colleague begins an intimate relationship with one of their patients. You become aware of the situation. How would you advise your PA colleague?

6. A 17 year old patient of yours comes to the office with unexplained bruises throughout their body. You suspect they may be abused by their significant other, but the patient denies it. What do you do?

7. A 15 year old patient of yours is requesting medical marijuana to help them deal with severe anxiety and PTSD and asks you not to tell their parents. What would you do?

8. An uninsured patient comes to the ER with abdominal pain. They need a CT scan of their abdomen but are refusing because they do not have the means to afford the scan. You know that without this scan, the patient may receive poor care and their medical condition could worsen. What would you do?

9. One of your PA school classmates has been posting concerning messages on social media, stating that they are misunderstood by society and feeling alone. In class, you notice that they do not regularly engage with classmates. What would you do?

10. A colleague makes a medical error that does not negatively impact the care of a patient. They ask that you not tell the patient when you see them for a follow up visit. How do you respond?

11. Your patient asks you about seeing a chiropractor or acupuncturist for their back pain. How do you advise them?

12. What are your thoughts on provider-assisted suicide?

CHAPTER 6: THE GROUP INTERVIEW

INTRODUCTION

The group interview is a common PA school interview tool that programs use to gauge how well you work with others and as a team. After all, one of the major tenants of the PA profession is teamwork, as PAs work with physicians, nurses, medical assistants, and other health professionals to comprehensively care for patients.

There are two major types of group interviews that programs utilize: The traditional group interview and the activity group interview.

TRADITIONAL GROUP INTERVIEW

In the traditional group interview, a group of applicants is interviewed by a single or multiple faculty members. Typically, a question is posed to the group and the applicants each take turns answering the question, sometimes building on the responses of other applicants. On occasion, the applicants may each be asked different questions as well. Thus, you may not get a chance to respond to each question that is asked.

There are some strategies to consider during the group interview. If a question is asked to the group, and you feel you have a good answer, it is in your best interest to be assertive and speak first. If you are not sure how to answer, you should let others speak while you formulate your response. You should use other applicant responses and build your response from their answers, but add your own uniqueness or personal insight to the question so that you aren't merely repeating back what another applicant has already said. Show some originality of thought. Alternatively, many questions will have more than one reasonable response, and you can thus use an alternative response that is different from other applicants.

During the group interview it is also important to develop rapport with the other applicants. Acknowledge their responses during your time to talk, and even credit them for a good response. Make sure you take time to speak and make your voice heard, but don't be overbearing and take up all of the time as this will reflect poorly on you especially if some applicants are not given a chance to speak.

Though any type of question can be asked in the group setting, most commonly the questions tend to be very open ended. For example, you might be asked about a challenge you've faced in your life or where you see the future of the PA profession heading in the next 10 years. There is plenty of opportunity for everyone to respond with these types of questions, so take your time and give them an answer they will remember!

ACTIVITY GROUP INTERVIEW

In this type of interview, interviewers may present the applicants with a hypothetical problem and require them to work together towards a solution. Applicants are again being judged by their ability to work as a team, as well as their problem-solving skills.

Do not make this into a competition with your group. Remember, some of the group members could be your future classmates, and PA school is all about working together with each other. Make sure to always stay composed. Do not raise your voice or argue. It is okay to disagree with group members, as long as it is done in a respectful manner.

One strategy would be to be the leader in the group. In this role you should facilitate discussion amongst the applicants and summarize as you go. Make sure that you take into consideration everyone's opinions and try to achieve consensus.

If you do not want to lead, you can simply be a valuable group member. Make sure you contribute in some way to the activity by engaging the other group members and trying to problem solve. Show how well you can communicate with others, and that you have your own opinions.

ACTIVITY EXAMPLES

Case Study Discussion:
Participants are given a medical case to read and discuss collectively. They may be asked to formulate a diagnosis, treatment plan, and discuss potential ethical considerations.

Role-playing Scenarios:
Applicants may be assigned different roles in a healthcare scenario and asked to act out how they would handle specific situations. This can assess interpersonal skills and the ability to work in a team.

Group Problem-Solving:
Teams may be presented with a complex problem related to healthcare, and they are required to collaborate to find a solution. This could involve prioritizing tasks, allocating resources, or making decisions under time constraints.

Team-building Activities:
Engaging in team-building exercises can help assess how well applicants work together. This could include problem-solving challenges, trust-building activities, or activities that require effective communication.

Ethical Dilemmas:
Discussing ethical scenarios related to healthcare allows the interviewers to evaluate an applicant's ability to navigate challenging situations and make sound decisions.

Group Presentation:

Applicants may be given a topic related to healthcare or medical ethics and asked to prepare a short group presentation. This assesses communication skills, the ability to convey information effectively, and teamwork.

Debates:

Organizing a debate on a healthcare-related topic can help interviewers evaluate an applicant's ability to articulate their thoughts, consider different perspectives, and engage in constructive discussions.

Critical Thinking Exercises:

Providing applicants with a set of data, research findings, or a medical article and asking them to analyze and discuss the information collectively can assess critical thinking and analytical skills.

Patient Interaction Simulation:

Applicants might participate in a simulated patient interaction where they work together to gather information, assess the patient's condition, and develop a plan of care.

Group Interview with Observers:

Interviewers may observe how applicants interact during a group discussion without actively participating. This allows them to assess communication skills, leadership potential, and the ability to collaborate with others.

CHAPTER 7:
THE INTERVIEW
WRITING SAMPLE

INTRODUCTION:

Some programs utilize a writing sample during the interview process. The writing sample is utilized for several reasons. Firstly, they want to see if you can synthesize and analyze a situation, form an opinion, and articulate your thoughts. Secondly, they simply want to see if you are a competent writer. They know that many times personal statements and supplemental application responses are reviewed by essay editing services, family members, friends, advisors, and others. Thus, they want to see how well you can write in the moment, unassisted. Finally, they may use the essay as an ethical scenario that they would like you to respond to. This is to your benefit because it gives you a chance to really think about the scenario and put together your thoughts before responding, unlike a traditional interview where you may only have a few seconds to think about the scenario and reply. Overall, you should write enough to answer the question thoroughly, nothing more and nothing less.

WRITING SAMPLE EXAMPLES

If there is a writing sample as part of the interview process, it could take various forms. Here are some possibilities:

Standard Prompt:
You may be given a prompt related to healthcare, medical ethics, or a current healthcare issue. The goal is to assess your ability to articulate your thoughts in writing and communicate effectively.

Personal Statement Review:

In some cases, the interviewers might ask you to review and discuss your personal statement. This could involve explaining your motivation for pursuing a career as a physician assistant, highlighting experiences, and discussing your goals.

Critical Analysis:

You might be presented with a case study or a healthcare-related scenario and asked to provide a written analysis. This could assess your critical thinking skills, problem-solving abilities, and your understanding of medical ethics.

Communication Skills Assessment:

Writing samples could also be used to evaluate your written communication skills, which are crucial for healthcare professionals. You might be asked to write a patient education handout or explain a medical concept in writing.

Remember, if a writing sample is part of the PA school interview process, it is likely designed to evaluate skills such as critical thinking, communication, and professionalism. Be sure to prepare by reviewing common healthcare topics, staying informed about current healthcare issues, and practicing articulating your thoughts in a clear and concise manner.

CHAPTER 8: ASKING QUESTIONS

As you prepare for your Physician Assistant (PA) school interview, it's essential to recognize that the questions you ask are as significant as the ones you answer. You will be given an opportunity to ask questions you may have about the program to faculty members or students. This chapter is dedicated to guiding you through the art of asking thoughtful and strategic questions, showcasing your genuine interest in the program and your potential role as a PA.

THE PURPOSE OF ASKING QUESTIONS

Firstly, understand that the questions you pose during your PA school interview serve several purposes. They allow you to gather essential information about the program, demonstrate your knowledge, and convey your enthusiasm. Moreover, asking insightful questions can leave a lasting impression on the interviewers, showcasing your genuine interest in their institution.

GENERAL CONSIDERATIONS

Before delving into specific questions, keep these general considerations in mind:

RESEARCH THE PROGRAM:

Ensure you've thoroughly researched the PA program. Familiarize yourself with the curriculum, clinical opportunities, faculty, and any unique aspects that distinguish the program from others. You do not want to ask simple questions that can easily be answered by checking the program website.

PERSONALIZE YOUR QUESTIONS:

Tailor your questions based on the information you couldn't find through standard research. This demonstrates your genuine curiosity and goes beyond generic inquiries.

Example Questions

1. Can you elaborate on any unique aspects of your program's curriculum or teaching philosophy?

This question allows you to understand the program's approach to education and whether it aligns with your learning style**.**

2. How does your program place students for clinical rotations, and what types of clinical experiences are available for electives?

Gain insights into the practical, hands-on experiences offered, and assess whether they align with your career goals.

3. Can you provide more information about opportunities for research, community outreach, or involvement in professional organizations within the program?

This question showcases your interest in contributing to the program beyond the classroom and clinical settings.

4. How does the program support student-faculty relationships, and are there opportunities for mentorship?

Understanding the support structure within the program can influence your overall experience.

5. What resources are available for students who may need additional academic support or assistance?

This question shows your awareness of potential challenges and your proactive approach to addressing them.

6. How would you describe the sense of community among students within the program?

Understanding the dynamics of student relationships can provide insight into the overall environment.

7. Are there student-led organizations or extracurricular activities related to the PA profession?

This question demonstrates your interest in being an active and engaged member of the student community.

8. What is the timeline for admission decisions, and what are the next steps in the process?

This question shows your eagerness to stay informed and engaged in the admissions process.

9. What inter-professional opportunities are available for students?

This question shows that you are eager to work as part of a team, as well as learn from and interact with other professions.

In general, you should avoid asking questions regarding PANCE pass rates, attrition rates, or anything that could be seen as a potential negative about a program. You want to project excitement about the program and show the program not only that you are eager to attend, but also are confident in the quality of the program.

Asking thoughtful questions during your PA school interview is an opportunity to showcase your genuine interest and gather crucial information for your decision-making process. Approach the interview not just as an evaluation of your suitability for the program but also as a chance for you to evaluate whether the program aligns with your goals and aspirations. Remember, the questions you ask are a powerful tool in shaping the narrative of your candidacy.

CHAPTER 9: NAVIGATING THE POST-INTERVIEW PERIOD

Congratulations! You've successfully navigated the intense and challenging process of the Physician Assistant (PA) school interview. As you exhale a sigh of relief, it's essential to shift your focus to the critical steps that follow your interview. This chapter will guide you through what to do after your PA school interview, helping you maximize your chances of securing a coveted spot in your desired program.

REFLECT ON YOUR PERFORMANCE

Take some time to reflect on your interview. Consider the questions asked, your responses, and how well you conveyed your passion for the profession. Identify any areas where you think you could improve or topics you wish you had elaborated on more. Reflecting on your performance can be a valuable learning experience, preparing you for potential future interviews or discussions.

SEND THANK-YOU EMAILS

While sending a thank-you email may not increase your chances of getting accepted, it certainly does not hurt! We advise that you promptly send personalized thank-you emails to each person who interviewed you. Express your gratitude for the opportunity and reiterate your enthusiasm for the program. Be concise but specific about what you enjoyed during the interview and why you believe the program is an excellent fit for your goals. This not only demonstrates professionalism but also keeps you fresh in the minds of the interviewers.

UPDATE YOUR APPLICATION

If you have any notable achievements, experiences, or academic accomplishments since submitting your application, update the admissions office. This can include new certifications, relevant coursework, or additional healthcare experience gained. However, avoid bombarding them with unnecessary information; focus on what adds value to your candidacy.

PREPARE FOR WAITLIST OR FURTHER INTERVIEWS

Some programs may place candidates on a waitlist after interviews, while others may conduct multiple rounds of interviews. Be mentally prepared for either scenario. Continue staying informed about the program, as this knowledge can be beneficial during waitlist or subsequent interviews. If you're placed on a waitlist, consider sending a letter of intent expressing your continued interest in the program.

STAY INFORMED AND ENGAGED

Stay connected with the PA program by following their social media accounts, newsletters, or blogs. Attend any virtual events or information sessions they may host. This not only demonstrates your ongoing interest but also keeps you informed about any updates or changes in the admissions process.

PLAN FOR MULTIPLE OFFERS

If you're fortunate enough to receive multiple offers, carefully weigh your options. Consider program strengths, location, cost, and any unique aspects that align with your career goals. It's wise to contact current students or alumni for insights into their experiences. Notify programs of your decision promptly, keeping in mind any deadlines for acceptance.

REFLECT ON YOUR ALTERNATIVES

While waiting for decisions, consider alternatives and create a plan B. Think about potential gap-year activities that could enhance your skills or experiences. This proactive approach ensures that you're prepared for any outcome and can make the most of your time. Consider sending emails to schools that you were rejected from to elicit advice about weaknesses on your application or interview and how best to improve them for the next application cycle.

The post-interview period is a crucial time in the PA school admissions process. By reflecting on your performance, expressing gratitude, staying informed, and planning for various outcomes, you position yourself as a proactive and engaged candidate. Remember, the journey to becoming a PA is not just about the destination but also the steps you take along the way. Good luck!

CHAPTER 10: ADDITIONAL PRACTICE QUESTIONS

Utilize this list of practice questions to prepare for your PA school interview thoroughly. Remember, practicing your responses will not only enhance your ability to articulate your thoughts but will also boost your confidence when facing the actual interview. Take the time to reflect on each question, craft thoughtful responses, and consider conducting mock interviews with peers or mentors to refine your communication skills.

GENERAL INTERVIEW QUESTIONS

Tell us about yourself and what motivated you to pursue a career as a Physician Assistant?

What do you understand about the role of a PA, and how does it differ from other healthcare professions?

Describe a challenging situation you faced in a healthcare setting and how you handled it.

How do you stay updated on current trends and developments in the field of healthcare and medicine?

Discuss a healthcare issue that you feel passionately about and explain why it's significant.

ACADEMIC AND PROFESSIONAL BACKGROUND

Can you elaborate on your academic background and highlight any coursework that has prepared you for the PA program?

How have your professional experiences, such as clinical or research positions, influenced your decision to become a PA?

Describe a situation where you worked in a team, highlighting your role and the outcome of the collaboration.

How do you plan to balance the rigorous academic demands of PA school with your personal and professional responsibilities?

Discuss any experiences you've had working with diverse populations and how these experiences have shaped your worldview.

ETHICAL AND SITUATIONAL QUESTIONS

Describe a situation where you faced an ethical dilemma in a healthcare setting and how you resolved it.

How do you handle stress, and what strategies do you use to maintain your well-being during challenging situations?

If you were faced with a patient who was non-compliant with medical advice, how would you approach the situation?

Discuss a mistake or setback you've experienced in your academic or professional journey and what you learned from it.

How do you prioritize patient care, especially when faced with time constraints?

QUESTIONS ABOUT YOUR UNDERSTANDING OF THE PA PROFESSION

What role do you believe technology plays in modern healthcare, and how should PAs adapt to these changes?

How do you envision the collaboration between PAs and other healthcare professionals in a clinical setting?

Describe the significance of cultural competence in the practice of medicine and how it applies to the PA profession.

What challenges do you foresee for the future of healthcare, and how can PAs contribute to addressing these challenges?

Explain your understanding of the importance of lifelong learning for PAs and how you plan to stay updated in your career.

PROGRAM-SPECIFIC QUESTIONS

What attracted you to our PA program, and how do you see yourself contributing to our community?

Can you discuss any specific aspects of our program's curriculum or resources that align with your learning preferences?

How do you plan to make the most of the clinical experiences offered in our program?

What do you hope to achieve during your time in our PA program, and how will it contribute to your long-term goals?

If accepted, how do you plan to be an active and engaged member of our PA program community?

CHAPTER 11: PRACTICING FOR INTERVIEWS

INTRODUCTION:

Welcome to your mock interview for PA school. This practice session aims to simulate a real PA school interview experience, helping you refine your responses, communication skills, and overall interview performance. Remember to approach this exercise with a positive mindset and a commitment to improvement.

BEFORE THE MOCK INTERVIEW

REVIEW YOUR APPLICATION:

Familiarize yourself with your application materials, including your personal statement, resume, and experiences. Be ready to discuss any aspect of your application.

RESEARCH THE PROGRAM:

Revisit information about the PA program you are interviewing for. Understand its mission, values, curriculum, and any unique features.

CHOOSE A COMFORTABLE SETTING:

Find a quiet and well-lit space for the mock interview, free from distractions. Ensure a stable internet connection if conducting a virtual interview.

DURING THE MOCK INTERVIEW

DRESS PROFESSIONALLY:

Wear professional attire to simulate the actual interview environment. This helps create a mindset of professionalism and readiness.

MOCK INTERVIEW STRUCTURE:

The mock interview will consist of common PA school interview questions, including personal, behavioral, and program-specific inquiries.

INTERVIEWER ROLE:

If possible, enlist a friend, family member, or mentor to act as the interviewer. Provide them with a list of questions to ask during the mock interview.

USE A TIMER:

Set a timer for the overall interview duration and allocate specific time for each question. This mimics the time constraints of a real interview.

RECORD THE MOCK INTERVIEW:

If feasible, record the mock interview session. Reviewing the recording later allows you to identify areas for improvement in your responses, body language, and overall presentation.

SCORING THE MOCK INTERVIEW:

Have your interviewer score each of your responses to the interview questions. Score from 1 to 5 where 1 means needs improvement and 5 is an excellent response. Have your interviewer score non-verbal factors as well such as your body language, eye contact, and appearance.

SAMPLE MOCK INTERVIEW QUESTIONS:

PERSONAL QUESTIONS:

Why do you want to become a Physician Assistant?

Can you tell us about a challenging situation you faced and how you handled it?

Discuss a significant accomplishment or experience from your healthcare background.

BEHAVIORAL QUESTIONS:

Describe a situation where you had to work in a team to achieve a goal.

How do you handle stress and pressure in a fast-paced healthcare environment?

Share an example of a time when you had to adapt to unexpected changes.

PROGRAM-SPECIFIC QUESTIONS:

What attracted you to our PA program?

How do you see yourself contributing to our program and the PA profession?

Can you discuss any specific aspect of our curriculum that excites you?

ETHICAL SCENARIO:

Present a hypothetical ethical scenario related to healthcare and ask the interviewee to discuss their approach and decision-making process.

POST-MOCK INTERVIEW:

SELF-REFLECTION:

Reflect on your performance. What went well, and what areas can be improved? Consider your communication style, clarity of responses, and overall confidence.

FEEDBACK FROM THE INTERVIEWER:

Seek feedback from the interviewer on your responses, presentation, and any specific areas for improvement. Use this feedback constructively.

REVIEW THE RECORDING:

If recorded, review the mock interview recording. Take note of non-verbal cues, body language, and areas where you can enhance your delivery.

ADJUST AND PRACTICE:

Adjust your approach based on feedback and self-reflection. Continue to practice addressing common questions and refining your responses.

ADDITIONAL RESOURCES

Personal Statement Review:

We whole-heartedly recommend myPAResource for all your personal statement needs. They have helped thousands of applicants revise their personal statement and get accepted into PA school.

Visit their website at **myPAresource.com** for details about their essay reviews.

Mock-Interviews/PA Coaching:

The Posh PA (Michele Neskey) is your one stop shop for all pre-PA advising needs, as well as mock interviews. They have several wonderful PA coaches suited for any applicant, and have helped hundreds of students get into their dream schools.

Visit her website at **micheleneskey.com** or message her on **Instagram @michele.theposhpa.**

Find Your Perfect PA Program:

The Applicant's Manual of Physician Associate Programs 2024 (updated annually) is the premier resource for researching programs and finding the schools that best fit you!

Find it on **Amazon** or connect on **Instagram @paprogrammanual.**

Notes:

Notes:

Notes:

Notes:

Made in the USA
Middletown, DE
07 June 2025

76693820R00060